Where Neuropsychiatric Diseases Converge

Vincent Berry, M.S.

Contents

List of Figures 2

Introduction 3

Background 4

Statement of Methods 5

Dopamine Circuitry 5

    Nigrostriatal Pathway 5

    Mesocorticolimbic Pathway 7

Regulation of Dopamine 8

    Dopamine Synthesis 8

    Dopamine Receptors 11

Neuropsychiatric Disorders 13

    Addiction 13

    Parkinson's Disease 16

    Schizophrenia 18

Discussion 20

Conclusion 21

Figures & Tables 23

References 30

Vita 41

List of Figures

Figure 1: Nurr1 target proteins (Jacobs et al., 2009)..23

Figure 2: Nurr1, Pitx3 & HDACs (Jacobs et al., 2009).......................................23

Figure 3: Mesolimbic DA System (Luscher and Malenka, 2011).......................24

Figure 4: Epigenetic control in Addiction (Nestler, 2014)..................................24

Figure 5: Dopamine Synthesis (Daubner, 2011)...25

Figure 6: Nigrostriatal DA and Parkinson's (Obeso et al., 2000).......................25

Figure 7a: Nurr1 expression in PD (Rojas et al., 2012).....................................26

Figure 7b: TH expression in PD (Rojas et al., 2012)...26

Figure 8a: Protein expression in DJ-1$^{-/-}$ rats (Sun et al., 2013)...................27

Figure 8b: Protein expression in Pink1$^{-/-}$ rats (Sun et al., 2013)................28

Figure 9: TH levels in Schizophrenics (Howes et al., 2013)..............................29

Figure 10: tardive dyskinesia from APDs (Seeman and Tinazzi, 2013).............29

Introduction

The basal ganglia are a group of subcortical nuclei that carry out critical functions in motor control and higher cortical processes, including cognition, behavioral set, emotion, context and motivation. The neuroanatomical nature of the basal ganglia is intricate, involving a variety of interconnected neurons that are topographically organized forming cortical loops. Dopamine (DA) neurons originating from the midbrain play a critical role in modulating activity of these circuits, and slight perturbations in DA systems may result in dysfunctional motor activity or neuropsychiatric illnesses, such as Schizophrenia (SZ), Parkinson's disease (PD), or addiction. Thus, by investigating the mechanisms that regulate DA neurons and how individual circuits interact with one another neuropsychiatric disorders may be better understood. This review examines the neurobiological underpinnings concerning the regulation of synthesis, neurotransmission, and neuroplasticity taking place within the nigrostriatal (mesostriatal) and mesocorticolimbic DA systems. It is hypothesized that DA neurons in the mesocorticolimbic and nigrostriatal circuits are regulated by similar biomolecular mechanisms, which may be why multiple DA systems are affected in pathogenic situations. For the purposes of this review, SZ, PD and addiction are used as paradigms to examine the neurobiological changes that take place throughout the DA systems. Some of the cellular modifications caused by these disease states include altered size and shape of neuron cell bodies, distorted dendritic outgrowth, reduced levels of DA and tyrosine hydroxylase, down regulation of dopamine D2-type receptors, up-regulation of $GABA_A$ receptors, and altered expression of dopamine transporter (DAT) and vesicular monoamine transporter (VMAT2). By examining the genetic and epigenetic changes that take place throughout DA neurons of the basal ganglia we may better understand how to treat and prevent neuropsychiatric illnesses.

Background

Dopamine is a neurotransmitter synthesized from the amino acid tyrosine in the nervous system. It is synthesized and stored in the nerve terminal where it resides within small, clear synaptic vesicles. Upon stimulation of DA producing neurons, intracellular Ca^{2+} concentrations increase to mediate DA release into the synaptic cleft. DA can then bind pre- and post-synaptically to produce its effects. The dopamine transporter (DAT) is then responsible for removing DA from the synaptic cleft and bringing it back into the presynaptic cell, whereby it can either be metabolized by monoamine oxidase (MAO) or repackaged into vesicles by vesicular monoamine transporter 2 (VMAT2) for further release.

DA neurons account for less than one percent of all brain cells and most of these neurons have their cell bodies situated in either the substantia nigra pars compacta (SNc) or ventral tegmental area (VTA) of the mesencephalon. The neurotransmitter is involved in many brain processes including motivation, reward, and motor control. Furthermore, the neurocircuitry of DA systems is intricate and very sensitive to distress, which often manifests serious neuropsychiatric illnesses. There is much to be learned about the etiology of neuropsychiatric as well as neurologic disorders and potential ways to treat them. Although different DA pathways are affected in Parkinson's disease (PD), Schizophrenia (SZ) and drug addiction, each of these disorders may be marked by similar biomolecular changes that are responsible for regulating DA activity. Thus, an understanding of all the DA pathways and how they interact may be useful to our understanding of neuropsychiatry. Because these systems are interrelated, it is hypothesized that genetic or epigenetic modifications that take place in one DA system may also influence the activity of other DA systems. That is, neuropathological conditions in one DA system may cause dysfunctions in another DA system.

Statement of Methods

This critical review outlines the findings of current and past neurobiological research focusing on the regulation and control of mesolimbic, mesocortical and nigrostriatal DA systems. Studies detailing the mechanisms that underlie dopamine regulation throughout the brain are used to illustrate how dopaminergic pathways may interact with one another, and how the regulation or dysregulation of one DA system may potentially lead to changes in other DA systems. In order to offer a thorough evaluation, research findings that both support and oppose the stated hypothesis are used throughout the review. Furthermore, the research methods of several studies are evaluated for any potential limitations they pose in scientific validity.

Dopamine Circuitry

Nigrostriatal Pathway

DA from the SNc excites neurons of the dorsal striatum (caudate nucleus and putamen) mediating signals in the nigrostriatal pathway, an important regulator of motor activities, behavior, decision-making, cognitive habits and learning (Fariello, 1979; Carli et al., 1985; 1989; Graybiel, 1997; Jog et al., 1999; Haber, 2003). Upon reaching the caudate-putamen, the circuit diverges into the direct- and indirect pathways, which have opposing functions (DeLong, 1990). Dopaminergic input from the SNc stimulates two classes of GABAergic medium spiny neurons (MSNs). Direct pathway (striatonigral) MSNs express dopamine D1 receptors, localize substance P and dynorphin, and ascend to the ventral pallidum (VP) and internal segment of the globus pallidus (GPi). GPi and SNr neurons then innervate the thalamus, yielding GABA-mediated inhibition. The circuit ends with thalamo-cortical glutamate projections that maintain the original topography of the circuit (Gerfen, 1992, Gong et al., 2003; Nicola, 2007). Thus, DA stimulation in the direct pathway ultimately leads to excitation of the cortex (Albin et al., 1989; Cepeda et al., 1993), allowing us to initiate and control body movements. This pathway also plays a role in reinforcement and reward seeking behavior (Gerfen, 1984, 1999; Albin et al., 1989; Bolam et al., 2000).

Alternatively, indirect pathway (striatopallidal) GABAergic MSNs express D2 dopamine receptors, localize enkephalin, and innervate GABA interneurons located in the globus pallidus external segment (GPe) and VP (Gerfen, 1992; Kawaguchi 1997; da Silva Lobo et al., 2006). GABA interneurons from the GPe project to the subthalmic nucleus (STN), which contains glutamate neurons that further extend to areas of the SNr and GPi. When striatopallidal MSNs are inactive, GPe neurons become disinhibited and release GABA onto STN cells, thereby preventing the release of glutamate in the GPi and SNr. This results in less GABA transmission to the thalamus, and therefore, more thalamo-cortical glutamate-mediated activation (disinhibition). These indirect pathway events are controlled by the inhibitory activity of D2 receptors expressed on striatopallidal MSNs, which when stimulated by DA, enhance downstream cortical activity (Bertran-Gonzalez et al. 2008; Smith and Villalba 2008). However, when striatopallidal MSNs are stimulated by cortical afferents the opposite occurs: downstream cerebral cortex activity is suppressed, which restricts voluntary movements, mediates aversion-type responses, and prevents reward sensations (Gerfen, 1984; Albin et al., 1989; Bolam et al., 2000; Haber et al., 2000; Voorn et al., 2004). The competing functions of the direct- and indirect pathways have important implications in Parkinson's disease (PD), which presents as neurodegeneration of nigrostriatal DA cells, causing regulatory disturbance and functional imbalance in the two pathways (Carlsson, 2002; Mallet et al., 2008; Wichmann & Dostrovsky, 2011).

Mesocorticolimbic Pathway

The mesocortical and mesolimbic systems both contain DA producing neurons with cell bodies that originate in the VTA, which is why they have often been grouped together as one circuit, the mesocorticolimbic pathway. However, this may be an oversimplification since each circuit has different target areas, and therefore, distinct functional activity. Midbrain VTA neurons of the mesolimbic system innervate several brain structures, including the nucleus accumbens (NAc), hippocampus, VP, amygdala, and prefrontal cortex (Fields et al., 2007; German & Manaye, 1993; Haber & Fudge, 1997). This pathway is the primary mediator of natural reinforcement and reward seeking behavior (Olds and Milner, 1954; Crow, 1973; Wise, 1978).

DA activation in the NAc is a common feature among abusive drugs and has been implicated in addictive disorders and compulsive behaviors (Kornetsky and Esposito, 1979; Salamone et al, 2007; Le Moal and Simon, 1991). Moreover, hyperactive DA is also the cause of positive symptoms associated with Schizophrenia (Van Rossum, 1966; Seeman et al., 1975; Carlsson, 1974; 1978; Snyder, 1972; Meltzer & Stahl, 1976). However, there has been disagreement as to whether the hyperactive state of this system may be attributed to excess presynaptic DA release and accumulation in the NAc of the ventral striatum (Meisenzahl et al., 2007; Lyon et al., 2011) or, if postsynaptic D2 receptors become overactive as a result of overexpression or increased affinity for the DA neurotransmitter (Van Rossum, 1966; Howes and Kapur, 2009; Lyon et al., 2011).

Mesocortical neurons are distinguished from mesolimbic ones in that they project to the cortex, specifically the medial prefrontal cortex (mPFC) and orbital frontal cortex (OFC). Each of these two areas can be divided further: the OFC includes the lateral, medial, dorsolateral, and ventral-orbital areas of the cortex, whereas the mPFC is primarily made up of the prelimbic, anterior cingulate, infralimbic and dorsal peduncular cortices (Groenewegen and Uylings, 2000; Robbins, 2000; Teffer and Semendeferi, 2012). Although principal pyramidal neurons in these cortical regions mainly express D1-like DA receptors with minor D2 receptor expression (Gaspar et al., 1995), GABA interneurons and presynaptic glutamatergic neurons have been shown to express both receptor subtypes to a similar extent (Sesack et al., 1995; Muly et al., 1998; Wedzony et al., 2001).

The executive functions mediated by the mesocortical system are consistent with the anatomical target areas and include working memory, attention, impulse control and cognitive flexibility. This system allows us to organize various biological stimuli and characterize them based on importance (salience), which ultimately results in the production of adaptive behaviors (Kelley and Berridge, 2002; Nesse and Berridge, 1997; Panksepp et al., 2002). Lesion studies have shown that the mPFC mainly mediates attention and set-shifting tasks (Birrell and Brown, 2000; Maddux and Holland, 2011; Floresco et al., 2008; McAlonan and Brown, 2003), whereas the OFC controls tasks related to reversal learning and response inhibition (Eagle et al., 2008; Chudasama et al., 2003; McAlonan and Brown, 2003). Hypoactive dopamine from the VTA to the dorsolateral and ventral-medial prefrontal cortical areas is hypothesized to underlie the negative cognitive and affective symptoms of Schizophrenia (Davidson et al., 2009; Sharma et al., 2006; Bowie et al., 2006), as well as the loss of self-control in addiction.

Regulation of Dopamine

Dopamine Synthesis

Dopamine synthesis begins with the amino acid phenylalanine, which is converted to tyrosine by the enzyme phenylalanine hydroxylase ([figure 5](#)). The rate-limiting step in DA synthesis is subsequent hydroxylation of tyrosine to form L-dihydroxyphenylalanine (L-DOPA). The enzyme tyrosine hydroxylase (TH) catalyzes this reaction and is required for DA and catecholamine synthesis (Nagatsu et al., 1964). Accordingly, TH expression is a major regulatory component in DA neurosynthesis, thus, the mechanisms that regulate TH expression may also be said to regulate DA expression. Dopamine is generated in the synaptic terminal when L-DOPA is decarboxylated by aromatic amino acid decarboxylase (AADC), an enzyme that may also serve to modulate DA levels, but does so trivially in comparison to TH. Nonetheless, control of TH is complex, involving both short- and long-term mechanisms at many different cellular levels. Regulation at the levels of transcription, translation, and epigenetic modification cause long-term genomic and proteomic changes, whereas phosphorylation and negative feedback by DA control the short-term effects of TH activity. It is important to note that the mechanisms controlling TH expression vary depending on the tissue, stage of development, and species (Kumer and Vrana, 1996). Understanding how TH is regulated is important, because changes in TH activity are thought to be involved in Schizophrenia and Parkinson's disease (Haavik and Toska, 1998).

At the level of gene expression, two important transcription factors have been shown to play a major role in regulating TH activity and dopamine neurotransmission: the nuclear receptor related 1 protein (Nurr1) and paired-like homeodomain transcription factor 3 (Pitx3) protein (Sakurada et al., 1999; Cazorla et al., 2000; Iwawaki et al., 2000; K.S. Kim et al., 2003; Martinat et al., 2006). Nurr1 is expressed in DA neurons of the mesencephalon during late stages of neuronal development, with levels peaking during terminal differentiation of DA cells (Volpicelli et al., 2004; Zetterström et al. 1997; Castillo et al. 1998). Research on Nurr1 function has largely involved animal models with null variants of Nurr1 alleles, and a majority of these experiments have demonstrated the role of Nurr1 in inducing TH gene expression, and thus, DA differentiation in neurons of the VTA and SNc (Zetterström et al. 1997; Castillo et al. 1998). Studies have also suggested that Nurr1 may be required for the survival and maintenance of DA levels in the midbrain (Saucedo-Cardenas et al., 1998; Eells et al., 2002). These conclusions were substantiated by the fact that Nurr1 knockout (Nurr1$^{-/-}$) mice had substantially reduced concentrations of TH protein in nigrostriatal and mesocorticolimbic DA neurons. However, norepinephrine (NE) levels in the striatum were unaffected in these studies (Saucedo-Cardenas et al., 1998), suggesting that other molecules or mechanisms may be involved (DA and TH are precursors to NE).

Jacobs et al. (2009) proposed a mechanism for Nurr1-mediated TH induction in mesencephalon-derived DA neurons that involves Pitx3, whereby both Pitx3 and Nurr1 were shown to induce TH expression by interacting with response elements in the upstream promoter region. In the absence of Pitx3 (Pitx3$^{-/-}$), the co-repressor SMRT (silencing mediator for retinoid or thyroid-hormone receptors) recruits histone deacetylases (HDACs), which repress the promoter region and prevent expression of the TH target gene (Huang et al., 2000; Guenther et al., 2001; Fischle et al., 2002). However, when Pitx3 is present, it causes the SMRT/HDAC complex to dissociate from Nurr1, thus, promoting transcription of the TH target gene (Jacobs et al., 2009). These findings were further supported by the use of HDAC inhibitors (i.e., sodium butyrate), which allowed the promoter region to remain acetylated, and therefore, active in the absence of Pitx3 (figure 2). In this way, Nurr1 and Pitx3 co-regulate TH at the transcriptional level. Additionally, Nurr1 has also been shown to regulate other genes necessary for DA neurotransmission through similar neurobiological mechanisms, including the genes that code for the dopamine transporter (DAT), vesicular monoamine transporter, and D2 receptor (Jankovic et al. 2005; Kadkhodaei et al. 2009), as depicted in figure 1. The roles of Nurr1 and Pitx3 in regulating dopaminergic neurons of the mesostriatal and mesocorticolimbic systems is more complicated in disease states and have implications for neuropsychiatric disorders.

A well-studied post-translational mechanism that regulates TH involves phosphorylation of the enzyme at different serine (Ser) residues, namely Ser40. Phosphorylation of Ser40 has been shown to increase TH activity by preventing downstream negative feedback by DA and other catecholamine products (Haycock et al., 1992; Sutherland et al., 1993). After catecholamines are synthesized, they feedback on TH to decrease the enzyme's V_{max} (Daubner et al. 1992). However, when Ser40 is phosphorylated, the affinity of [feedback] catecholamines for TH decreases (K_D increases), which allows TH to increase its activity (McCulloch et al., 2001; Sura et al., 2004). Phosphorylation of TH is mainly carried out by the actions of protein kinase A (PKA). Thus, PKA mediated signaling may also be involved in DA regulation.

Dopamine Receptors

Within the synaptic cleft, DA produces its effects primarily through two classes of metabotropic (GPCR) receptors: D1-like (D1 and D5) and D2-like (D2, D3, and D4) receptors (Missale et al., 1998). D1 receptors are bound to excitatory $G\alpha_s$ protein on the intracellular surface, which stimulates adenylyl cyclase, producing cAMP that mediates downstream signaling events. Conversely, D2 receptors are mainly inhibitory and function through $G\alpha_i$ protein on the G-protein complex (Missale et al., 1998). D1-type receptors are expressed post-synaptically on target cells, whereas D2 and D3 receptors of the D2-type are expressed both post-synaptically and presynaptically (autoreceptors) (Sokoloff et al., 2006; Rondou et al., 2010).

Furthermore, D1R/D2R heterodimers are coupled to $G\alpha_q$ and thereby control DAG/IP3 signaling (Lee et al., 2004). In examining DA regulation, however, the D2 receptor is of special concern.

The function of the D2 receptor varies depending on whether it is expressed on presynaptic or post-synaptic cells. Post-synaptic D2 excitation generally results in increased locomotor activity, whereas presynaptic D2 autoreceptor excitation results in decreased locomotor activity. Thus, D2 autoreceptors are a major regulatory component of DA and are involved in controlling the neurotransmitter's synthesis, release, and firing rate (Wolf and Roth, 1990; Missale et al., 1998). Nonetheless, D2 receptors also play a major role in addiction and Schizophrenia. Hyperactive mesolimbic D2 receptor activity mediates the positive symptoms of Schizophrenia; antipsychotic drugs exert their effects primarily by antagonizing the D2 receptor (Snyder et al., 1970; Roth et al., 2004). D2 receptor blockade is succeeded by a progressive increase in Nurr77 expression in D2R-expressing neurons (Beaudry et al., 2000; Sanchez et al., 2014). Experiments using transgenic mice, GFP, and antipsychotic drugs have helped document this occurrence in D2 MSNs of the striatopallidal pathway (Beaudry et al., 2000; Sanchez et al., 2014). In these neurons, Nur77 contributes to enkephalin expression through a DARPP32 associated mechanism (Ethier et al., 2004). Studies using $Nurr77^{-/-}$ transgenic mice showed that Nurr77 impacts Nurr1 and TH expression. Mice with the $Nurr77^{-/-}$ phenotype had significantly higher levels of Nurr1 mRNA in the SNc and VTA, and TH mRNA was also upregulated in the SNc (Gilbert et al. 2006). Moreover, TH activity and turnover is increased in Nurr77 deficient cells. Further support for the role of Nurr77 in controlling DA release was noted when haloperidol administration reduced levels of DA in $Nurr77^{+/+}$ mice, but had no effect on DA levels in $Nurr77^{-/-}$ mice (Gilbert et al. 2006).

Neuropsychiatric Disorders

Addiction

Addiction is a physiological event marked by synaptic changes throughout the mesocorticolimbic DA system (Wise et al., 1987; Koob, 1992). As depicted in figure 3, all drugs of abuse work acutely to release excessive amounts of DA from VTA neurons, especially ones that project to the NAc (Di-Chiara and Imperato, 1988; Nestler, 2005). This event, however, can be mediated through several different mechanisms. For example, cocaine accomplishes this task by inhibiting the dopamine transporter (DAT) and preventing DA reuptake into the presynaptic cell, whereas opioids inhibit GABAergic interneurons and, in turn, disinhibit VTA DA neurons. Chronic exposure to cocaine and other drugs of abuse causes structural changes in VTA and NAc neurons. Specifically, VTA cell bodies decrease in size (Nestler, 2005; Sklair-Tavron et al., 1996) and NAc DA neurons expand their dendrites to areas of the prefrontal cortex (Robinson and Kolb, 2004; Brown and Kolb, 2001; McDonald et al., 2005; Robinson et al., 2001). Furthermore, when drug administration ceases in an addicted individual, basal DA firing from the VTA decreases substantially (Pierce and Kalivas, 1997). Also important to note is the downregulation of post-synaptic D2 receptor expression in the ventral striatum of cocaine users (Volkow et al., 2007). The probable explanation is that the system is reflexively compensating for excess DA.

PET brain imaging studies have shown that drug addiction results in decreased activity of mesocorticolimbic DAergic neurons projecting to the dorsolateral prefrontal cortex (DLPFC), orbitofrontal cortex (OFC) and anterior cingulate gyrus (ACG) (London et al., 1990; Volkow et al., 2007). The lack of stimulation to these cortical areas may be attributed to the decrease of D2 receptors in the striatum, a result of excess DA. This hypothesis is supported by experiments using rodents overexpressing D2R in the NAc. Rats overexpressing D2R reduced self-administration of alcohol compared to control rats and those underexpressing D2R (Thanos et al., 2001). Furthermore, people with a family history of alcoholism who had not developed alcoholism had significantly greater expression of D2R in the NAc as compared to people with no family history of alcoholism (Volkow et al., 2006). Under normal physiologic conditions, the DLPFC, OFC and ACG exert inhibitory behavioral control (Goldstein and Volkow, 2002) and consistent emotional states (Phan et al., 2002) that depend on excitatory input from the NAc. Thus, a lack of transmission from the NAc to these areas due to reduced NAc D2R stimulation is thought to facilitate the loss of self-control in addicted subjects (Volkow et al., 2009). The hippocampus and amygdala also play important roles in memory and emotion, respectively, adding yet another layer of complexity to drug reinforcement and reward seeking behavior (Volkow et al., 2009). Thus, a mechanism by which disturbances in one DA system cause changes in another is observed in the process of addiction.

An important question to ask is, "Given similar circumstances and drug exposure, why do some individuals become addicted and not others?" The answer may lie in the action of D2 receptors that influence cortical areas responsible for salience and self-control. Some researchers have proposed that neurophysiological changes take place early in life and certain environmental factors alter the structure of mesocorticolimbic neurons. For example, it has been suggested that children neglected by their parents may be more vulnerable to drug abuse later in life (De Bellis, 2002). It was further proposed that neglected children have increased enzymatic activity of dopamine beta hydroxylase (De Bellis, 2002), the protein that catalyzes the conversion of DA to norepinephrine. If true, this would lead to decreased D2R activity during developmental stages of the brain, and may make an individual more susceptible to addiction as a means to compensate for less D2 stimulation. However, the reported study did not follow this cohort to support such an interpretation.

Of concern is the impact that drug exposure has on the epigenetic landscape of DA systems. Chronic cocaine administration has been shown to both increase and decrease histone 3 and histone 4 (H3 and H4) acetylation in the NAc by histone acetyl transferases (HATs), CREB binding protein (CBP) and class II histone deacetylases (HDACs) resulting in short and long term changes that oppose each other (Renthal et al., 2007; Malvaez et al., 2011; Taniguchi et al., 2012). H4 acetylation has been shown to increase during acute cocaine exposure but doesn't change during chronic exposure, because the chronic condition desensitizes cFOS expression (Kumar et al., 2005; Renthal et al., 2008). Conversely, BDNF and Cdk5 promoters show H3 acetylation only after chronic cocaine exposure—consistent with the induction of these genes after chronic exposure. In general, hyperacetylation results in increased expression of genes and hypoacetylation decreases expression. However, in the larger context of epigenetic modification, acetylation contributes minimally compared to the effects of methylation, i.e., methylation sustains changes in gene expression, whereas acetylation is more complicated and time-dependent.

The histone methyltransferases (HMTs) G9a and G9a-like protein (GLP) decrease in number in the NAc following chronic cocaine exposure. This decrease potentiates drug response by increasing dendritic outgrowth of NAc neurons to DLPFC, OFC and ACG (Maze et al., 2010). The result is enhanced synaptic plasticity associated with addiction. Moreover, by changing the chromatin structure, G9a opposes ΔFosB induction, an important transcription factor involved in the addictive process (Robison and Nestler, 2011). H3K9me2 usually binds to the ΔFosB promoter region to block gene transcription of the $GABA_A$ receptor (Maze et al.,

2010; Sun et al., 2012). By methylating H3K9 (lysine residue 9 on histone 3) and thereby forming H3K9me2, G9a indirectly blocks $GABA_A$ transcription. However, G9a concentration diminishes during chronic cocaine administration, and so H3K9 remains unmethylated and ΔFosB is free to induce $GABA_A$ transcription in the NAc. Ultimately, this results in increased inhibitory tone in the NAc and frontal areas of the cortex (Maze et al., 2010; Sun et al., 2012). Paradoxically, G9a expression is later induced by chronic exposure, a result of prolonged HDAC inhibition from increased $GABA_A$ stimulation, which explains the opposing attenuation and stimulation effects of this intricate mechanism (figure 4). We must note that this is only one of several possible mechanisms responsible for controlling epigenetic modification in mesocorticolimbic DA neurons. Research in this area is still expanding, and almost all the studies to date focus on the role of lysine in controlling promoter activity. Clearly, research in this area should recognize the involvement of other amino acids in epigenetic modification. Future research in this area should include genome-wide mapping and other amino acids.

Parkinson's Disease

Parkinson's disease is a neurodegenerative disorder that presents as a loss of DAergic input from the SNc to the striatum. As a result, the direct pathway becomes underactive and the indirect pathway becomes overactive, which ultimately inhibits thalamo-cortical neurons that facilitate motor control (figure 6). The motor symptoms associated with this mechanism are rigidity, tremor, bradykinesia and postural instability. Some studies have proposed that alterations in Nurr1 expression may be a risk factor for PD (Jankovic et al., 2005). In PD, α-synuclein containing neurons in the SNc have been shown to contain substantially lower levels of Nurr1 (Beaudry et al., 2000) and, by extension, decreased expression of TH and DA.

Furthermore, MPTP (1-methyl-4-phenyl-1,2,3,6-tetrahydropyridine)-induced neurotoxicity results in Parkinson-like symptoms. This model has been used to detect significant reductions in Nurr1, Pitx3, and TH expression (Rojas et al., 2012) ([figures 7a and 7b](#)). This ultimately impacts expression of striatal D2R, VMAT2, DAT, and TH (Rojas et al., 2012)—also observed in addiction. Dendritic spines extending from MSNs in the striatum also undergo biochemical changes that cause them to decrease in number. DA in the nigrostriatal system is normally responsible for regulating glutamate input from the cortex and GABAergic output in the striatum, so when DA neurons degenerate in PD, the distribution of NMDA & AMPA receptors on MSNs changes to compensate for the disruption (Dunah et all., 2000). This further alters the excitatory state of neurons in this system, which impacts motor control downstream.

Although the mechanisms of DA regulation are very similar in PD and addiction, the interactions between Nurr1 and PD-related genes is quite complicated. Deng et al. (2008) suppressed Nurr1 expression in vitro using siRNA interference. As expected, they observed significant reductions in mRNA of DA-related proteins that Nurr1 normally induces (D2R, TH, DAT, and VMAT2). However, they also found major increases in PINK1 (~70%) and α-synuclein (25%), two genes associated with PD. Another recent study by Sun et al. (2013) used knockout rats lacking DJ-1 and Pink1 genes to study the effect of PD-related genes on DA-related protein. They verified the findings of previous experiments showing that D2 receptors are upregulated in the striatum of DJ-1$^{-/-}$ and Pink1$^{-/-}$ rats ([figures 8a and 8b](#)) and D1 receptors are only expressed in greater amounts in DJ-1 knockout rats. They also found that DAT expression was unaffected by the lack of DJ-1 and Pink1, whereas VMAT2 expression was only slightly greater in DJ-1 null rats. Findings by Rousseaux et al. (2012) using DJ-1$^{-/-}$ mice revealed increased levels of ΔFosB, which is upregulated in striatal neurons expressing D2R. As seen in other DA systems, the altered expression of dopamine receptors and other DA-related proteins in the striatum may represent a regulatory mechanism that compensates for DA loss from the SNc. However, more work is needed to describe the mechanisms involved in DAergic gene interaction with PD-related genes.

Schizophrenia

Schizophrenia is a complicated neuropsychiatric disorder marked by positive and negative symptoms that result from perturbations in the mesocorticolimbic DA system. Positive symptoms include psychosis (hallucinations, delusions and illusions) and disrupted flow of ideas (thought disorder). Negative and cognitive symptoms include deficits in attention, memory loss, reduced executive function, apathy, distorted speech, anhedonia, and social withdrawal. In general, positive symptoms are due to overactivation of D2 receptors in the NAc of the mesolimbic system, as well as overactivation of serotonin $5HT_{2A}$ receptors. Negative and cognitive symptoms are attributed to underactive D1 receptor stimulation in the prefrontal cortex of the mesocortical pathway (Davis et al., 1991). The current model of SZ holds that negative symptoms in the prodromal stage increase progressively, leading to psychotic episodes and positive symptoms in the mid-to-late phase. However, a causal relationship between hypoactive mesocortical DA neurons and hyperactivity in mesolimbic ones has not been established. This makes it difficult to comprehend the underlying etiology and ways to treat it.

In the past, there has been disagreement as to whether the hyperactive state of the mesolimbic system is attributed to excess presynaptic DA release in the striatum (Howes et al., 2007; Meisenzahl et al., 2007; Lyon et al., 2011), or overactivity of postsynaptic D2 receptors resulting from overexpression and/or increased affinity for DA (Howes and Kapur, 2009; Lyon et al., 2011). With the use of PET studies it is now generally accepted that the former is responsible (Shotbolt et al., 2011; Demjaha et al., 2012). Post-mortem studies of patients with SZ have shown that the expression and activity of TH is altered in the SNc (Howes et al., 2013) (figure 9). This may suggest yet another mechanism of DA regulation in common with other disease states. However, studies have shown that only 1% of patients with SZ have mutations in Nurr1, indicating that this regulatory mechanism probably does not underlie the etiology of SZ.

One might then ask what the origin of the overactive DA neurons is. The ventral hippocampus (vHipp) sends glutamate projections to the NAc, wherein extrinsic GABAergic neurons synapse on GABAergic neurons of the ventral pallidum. Fibers from these GABAergic neurons of the ventral pallidum descend to the VTA to constrain DA release. In SZ, the glutamatergic pathway from vHipp to NAc is overactive, so it enhances GABA signaling from the NAc to the pallidum, which in turn inhibits the GABA pathway from pallidum to VTA. Ultimately, this disinhibits DA neurons in the VTA, enhancing its messaging to the NAc. However, we do not yet understand the increased glutamate release from cells in the vHipp.

As previously described, antipsychotic drugs antagonize the D2 receptor to attenuate the positive symptoms. The subsequent rise in Nurr77 may attenuate TH and DA synthesis in the long run. Research has suggested that SZ patients using antipsychotic drugs are more likely to develop tardive dyskinesia (Tinazzi et al., 2012), raising the possibility of another interaction between the limbic and motor DA systems. The proposed mechanism by which this process occurs is briefly outlined in figure 10. The antipsychotic Aripiprazole, however, is a partial agonist at D2 receptors with much greater affinity than DA for the receptor. Thus, when Aripiprazole is administered, DA doesn't bind to D2R and the positive symptoms are reduced.

Discussion

Mesocorticolimbic and nigrostriatal DA systems have similar mechanisms that regulate DA synthesis, release, reuptake, and storage. Their overlapping activity is a consequence of their interconnected anatomy and regulatory mechanisms, possibly explaining why altered activity in one system may lead to changes in the other. As hypothesized, the two DA systems have analogous mechanisms of regulation, which involve similar transcription factors (Nurr1, Nurr77 and Pitx3) responsible for DA and DA-like protein expression. However, the evidence to date does not support the idea that converging biomolecular mechanisms of DA regulation play a role in dysfunctional states, as in neuropsychiatric disorders. Indeed, it appears that the biomolecular mechanisms involved in hyperactive mesolimbic DA in addiction are fundamentally different from those responsible for excess mesolimbic DA in schizophrenia.

Nonetheless, a common feature among the neuropsychiatric disorders described is altered structure and function of DA neurons in the striatum. The altered expression of the DA neurotransmitter, its receptors, and other DA-related proteins in the striatum are thought to be regulatory processes that attempt to compensate for changes in DA activity. For example, D2R dysfunction has been shown to result in greater quantities of Nurr1 mRNA, thus, greater concentrations of DA in the SNc. Another possible explanation is that D2R dysfunction occurs both pre- and post-synaptically, and so D2 autoreceptor dysfunction on presynaptic cells results in greater [unregulated] concentrations of DA (Tseng et al., 2000). However, the nature of scientific experimentation as well as the complexity of the systems being examined makes it nearly impossible to deduce causal relationships. Nonetheless, we can hypothesize and make inductive claims with high levels of confidence as to the factors that may be at play. With this in mind, the similarities and differences among DA neurons in different disease states are complex and require more investigation.

Conclusion

The basal ganglia are key sites of DAergic neurotransmission and have roles in cognition, behavioral set, emotion, context and motivation. Because the neuroanatomy of the basal nuclei is structured such that they communicate with several areas of the brain, they often have overlapping activities. Changes in DA and DA-related protein expression throughout the basal nuclei often result in altered motor activity and/or behavior, as seen in Schizophrenia, Parkinson's disease, and addiction. Thus, by understanding how DA is controlled throughout the brain, neuropsychiatric disorders may be better be understood.

Alterations in one DA system are often accompanied by disturbances in another DA system. This supports the idea that disturbances in different DA systems may be directly related to each other. Nonetheless, the idea that changes in different DA systems occur as para-phenomena without any causal relationships also withstands criticism under such circumstances, since different DA systems are disturbed through a variety of neurobiological mechanisms. That is, there is not a common neuropathological process that takes place between the different DA systems in various disease states, at least not at the molecular level. However, it is important to note that the mechanisms of DA regulation discussed in this review are only a select few. There are several other molecular mechanisms that control DAergic activity that are not discussed in this review and which may involve a commonality among the different DA circuits.

The neurocircuitry of DA systems throughout the brain have been studied and mapped out thoroughly. The three DA systems form loops, which often involve cortical afferents and efferents to and from the midbrain, respectively. However, since the DA circuits involve loops, the origin and source of regulation are difficult to extricate. Although the focus of this review was regulation of DA networks as they originate from the mesencephalon, other researchers propose a "top-down" approach involving projections that begin in the cortex. This is important for purposes of elucidating the etiology of neuropsychiatric diseases. If the origin of unregulated DA varies in different neuropsychiatric diseases and DA circuits, then this would also provide support for the idea that the three DA systems are regulated differently. Indeed, the origin of dysregulated DA in SZ (cortex) is different than in PD (SNc). Thus, a more thorough investigation would integrate the model used in this review with the "top-down" approach.

Dopamine is a complex neurotransmitter involved in many different processes. The neurobiological mechanisms that regulate its synthesis, release, and actions on other neurons are multifaceted and require more investigation. Future research should be directed toward understanding genetic and epigenetic changes that result in dysfunctional DA states. Furthermore, genome-wide mapping of different genes in disease states and their relationship(s) to genes involved in DA transmission need to be further examined.

Figures & Tables

Figure 1 (Jacobs et al., 2009)

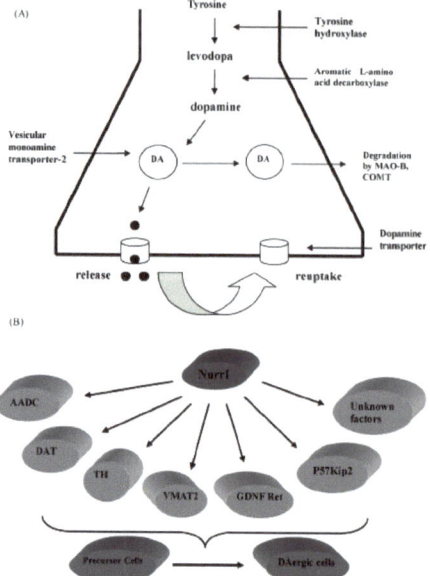

Fig. 4. Nurr1 regulates expression of AADC, DAT, TH, VMAT-2 Ret and P57Kip2 that are essential in DAergic phenotype and functional maintenance. (A) Shows the process of synthesis of dopamine. TH and AADC are critical enzymes for biosynthesis of dopamine. VMAT-2 participates in the storage of dopamine and DAT takes part in reuptake of dopamine. (B) Introduction of AADC, DAT, GDNF Ret, TH, P57Kip2, VMAT-2 and other unknown factors in mensencephalic DA neurons requires Nurr1.

Figure 2 (Jacobs et al., 2009)

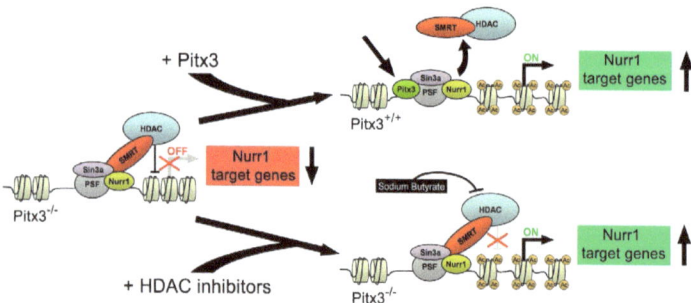

Figure 3 (Luscher and Malenka, 2011)

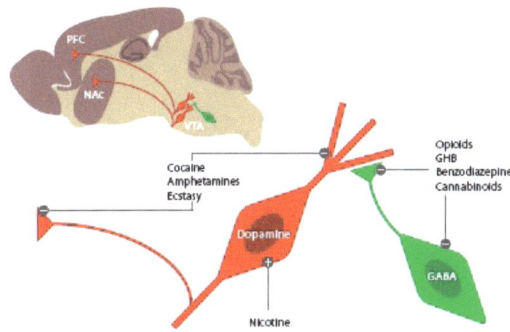

Figure 4 (Nestler, 2014)

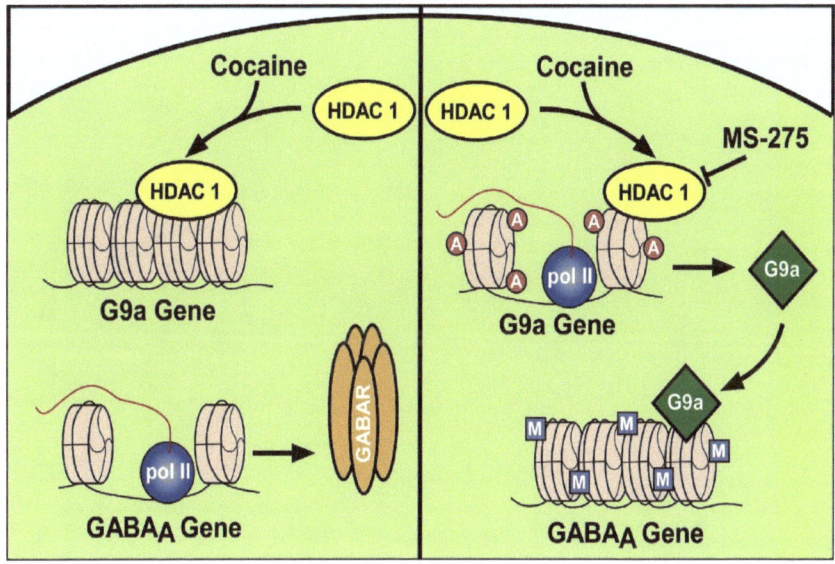

Figure 5 (Daubner, 2011)

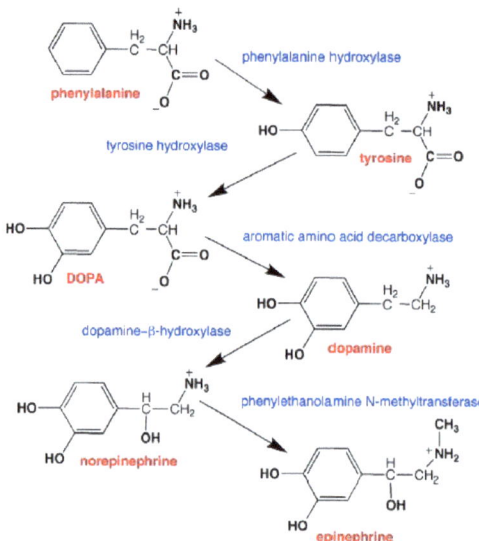

Fig. 1. The biosynthetic pathway for the catecholamine neurotransmitters. Phenylalanine hydroxylase converts phenylalanine to tyrosine, tyrosine hydroxylase hydroxylates tyrosine to L-DOPA. DOPA is converted to dopamine by aromatic amino acid decarboxylase. Dopamine-β-hydroxylase hydroxylates dopamine to norepinephrine, which is methylated to epinephrine by phenylethanolamine N-methyltransferase. Tyrosine hydroxylase is the rate-limiting enzyme of the pathway.

Figure 6 (Obeso et al., 2000)

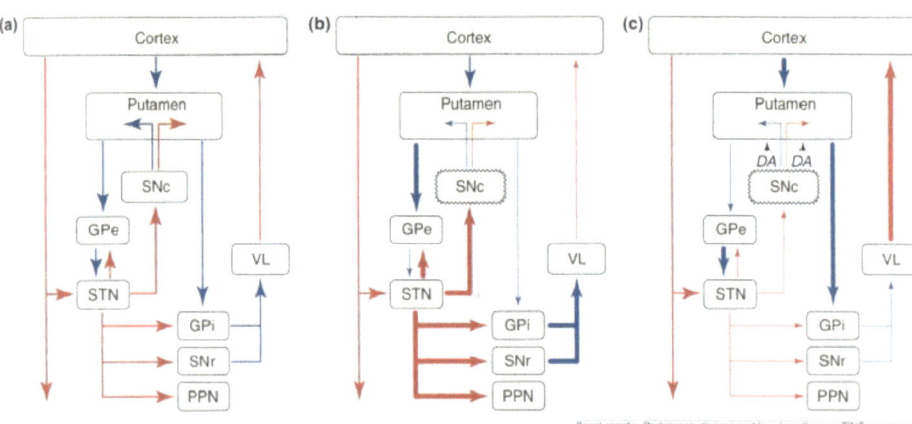

Fig. 1. Schematic of the classic model of the basal ganglia. The (a) normal, (b) parkinsonian and (c) dyskinetic states are depicted. Blue arrows indicate inhibitory projections and red arrows represent excitatory projections. The thickness of the arrows indicates the degree of activation of each projection. Note that the striatum communicates with output neurons in the globus pallidus pars interna (GPi) and substantia nigra pars reticularis (SNr) through a direct pathway, and with synaptic connections in the globus pallidus pars externa (GPe) and the subthalamic nucleus (STN) through an indirect pathway. Dopamine is thought to inhibit neuronal activity in the indirect pathway and to excite neurons in the direct pathway. (b) In the parkinsonian state, dopamine depletion leads to disinhibition of dopamine D2-receptor-bearing striatal neurons in the indirect pathway leading to increased inhibition of the GPe, and disinhibition of the STN. The resulting overactivity in STN neurons leads to excess excitation of neurons in the GPi/SNr and overinhibition of thalamo-cortical and brainstem motor centers resulting in parkinsonism. (c) Dyskinesia induced by L-dopa is characterized by reduced activity in the STN. The classical model proposes that this is due to dopamine-induced overinhibition of striato-GPe neurons, resulting in excess inhibition of the STN and reduced activation of GPi/SNr. The net result is reduced inhibition of thalamo-cortical neurons with excess drive of cortical motor areas resulting in dyskinesia. Abbreviations: DA, dopamine; PPN, pedunculopontine nuclei; SNc, substantia nigra pars compacta; VL, ventralis lateralis. Reproduced with permission from Ref. 7.

Figure 7a (Rojas et al., 2012)

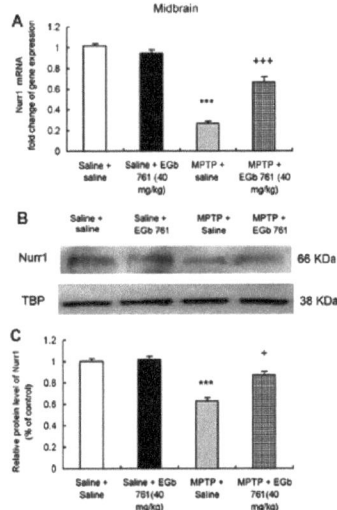

Fig. 3. Upregulation of Nurr1 gene expression and protein levels by EGb 761 against MPTP-induced neurotoxicity in the midbrain. (A) Relative levels of Nurr1 mRNA were analyzed by qPCR. The expression levels were normalized using the GAPDH gene. The results are reported as fold change compared to the control group (saline + saline) of 6–8 animals per group. (B) Representative Western blot of Nurr1 and TBP proteins. (C) Densitometric analysis of Western blot of Nurr1 protein levels in midbrain compared to TBP protein (n = 4 mice per group). Data are expressed as the mean ± SEM. Differences were analyzed with one-way ANOVA followed by post hoc Duncan's tests. ***$p < 0.001$ compared to the "saline + saline" group; +$P < 0.05$ and +++$P < 0.001$ compared to the "MPTP + saline" group. TBP, TATA box-binding protein; MPTP, 1-Methyl-4-phenyl-1,2,3,6-tetrahydropyridine; EGb 761, Ginkgo biloba extract.

Figure 7b (Rojas et al., 2012)

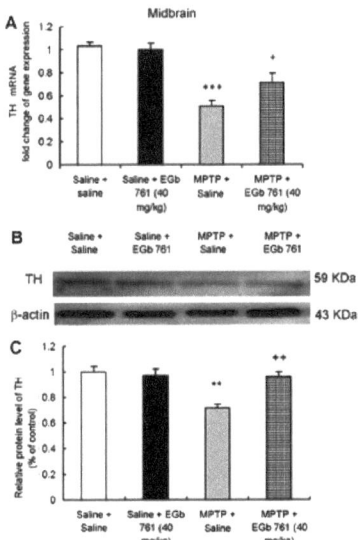

Fig. 1. EGb 761 upregulates Th mRNA and protein levels against the dopaminergic neurotoxicity induced by MPTP in the midbrain. (A) Relative Th mRNA levels were analyzed by qPCR. The expression levels were normalized to the GAPDH gene. The results are expressed as fold change compared to the control group (saline + saline) of 6–8 animals per group. (B) Representative Western blot of Th and β-actin (C) Densitometric analysis of Western blot of Th protein levels in midbrain compared to β-actin (n = 4 animals per group). Data are expressed as the mean ± SEM. Differences were analyzed with a one-way ANOVA followed by post hoc Duncan's tests **$P < 0.01$ and ***$P < 0.001$ compared to the "saline + saline" group; +$P < 0.05$ and ++$P < 0.01$ compared to the "MPTP + saline" group. MPTP, 1-Methyl-4-phenyl-1,2,3,6-tetrahydropyridine; EGb 761, Ginkgo biloba extract.

Figure 8a (Sun et al., 2013)

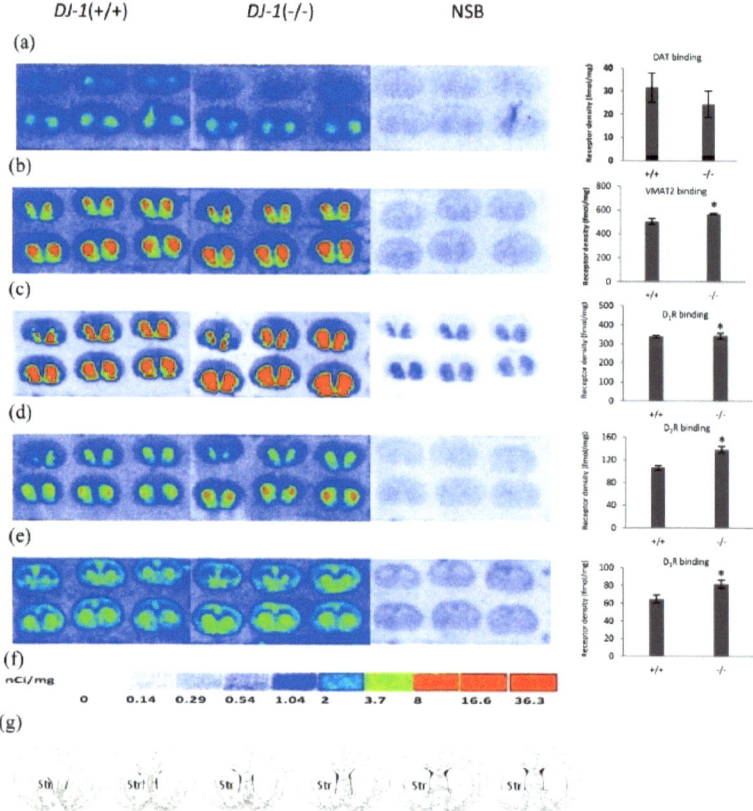

Fig. 1. Quantitative autoradiographic analysis of DAT, DTBZ and dopamine receptors densities in the *DJ-1* gene knockout rat models of PD. Autoradiograms show binding of 8.5 nM [^{3}H]WIN35428 (a), 23.5 nM [^{3}H]DTBZ (b), 3.8 nM [^{3}H]SCH23390 (c), 4.4 nM [^{3}H]raclopride (d) and 5.9 nM [^{3}H]**WC-10** (e) on multiple brain sections through the striatum in the *DJ-1* gene knockout and wild-type littermate rat. Nonspecific binding was determined in the presence of 1 μM nomifensine (for [^{3}H]WIN35428), 1 μM *S*(−)-tetrabenazine (for [^{3}H]DTBZ), 1 μM (+) butaclamol (for [^{3}H]SCH23390), 1 μM *S*(−)-eticlopride (for [^{3}H]raclopride and [^{3}H]**WC-10**). DAT binding did not significantly change in *DJ-1* gene knockout rat (a). The densities of VMAT2, dopamine D_1, D_2 and D_3 receptors were significantly increased in *DJ-1* gene knockout rats (b–e). [^{3}H]Microscale standards (ranging from 0 to 36.3 nCi/mg) were also counted (f). Schematic rat brain sections showing the rostral to caudal extent of the striatum, the region of interest in which DAT, VMAT2, D_1, D_2, and D_3 receptors were quantified, across a total of six sections (g). NSB, nonspecific binding; Str, striatum. *$p < 0.05$ for *DJ-1* knockout rat vs. control rat.

Figure 8b (Sun et al., 2013)

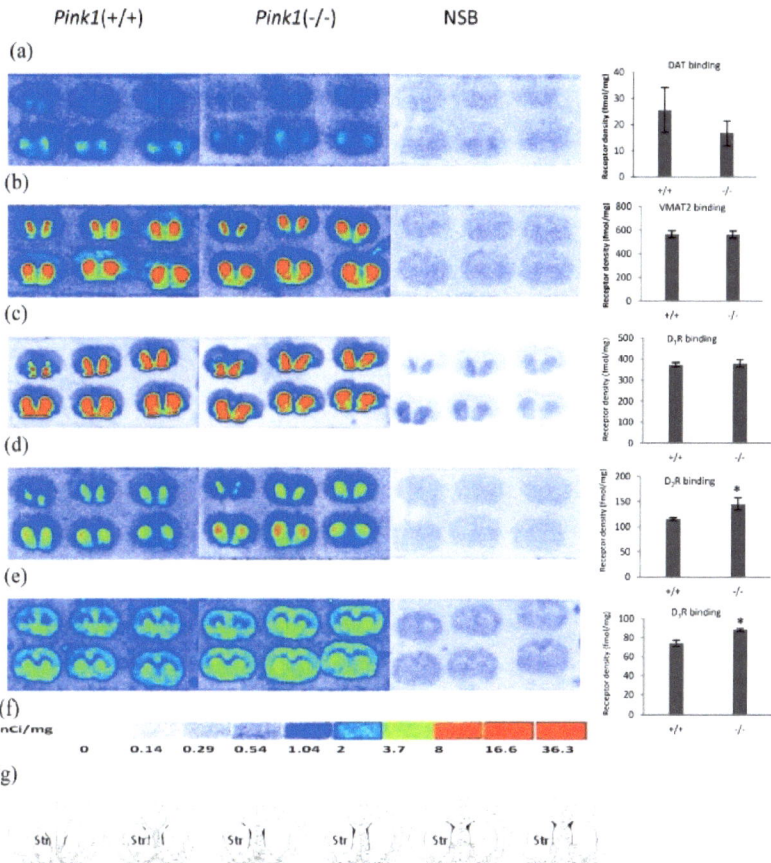

Fig. 2. Quantitative autoradiographic analysis of DAT, DTBZ and dopamine receptors densities in the *PINK1* gene knockout rat models of PD. Autoradiograms show binding of 8.5 nM [^{3}H]WIN35428 (a), 23.5 nM [^{3}H]DTBZ (b), 3.8 nM [^{3}H]SCH23390 (c), 4.4 nM [^{3}H]raclopride (d) and 5.9 nM [^{3}H]WC-10 (e) on multiple brain sections through the striatum in the *PINK1* gene knockout and wild-type littermate rat. Nonspecific binding was determined in presence of 1 μM nomifensine (for [^{3}H]WIN35428), 1 μM S(−)-tetrabenazine (for [^{3}H]DTBZ), 1 μM (+) butaclamol (for [^{3}H]SCH23390), 1 μM S(−)-eticlopride (for [^{3}H]raclopride and [^{3}H]WC-10). DAT, VMAT2 and D$_1$ receptor binding did not change in *PINK1* gene knockout rat (a–c). The densities of dopamine D$_2$ and D$_3$ receptors were significant upregulated in *PINK1* gene knockout rats (d and e). [^{3}H]Microscale standards (ranging from 0 to 36.3 nCi/mg) were also counted (f). Schematic rat brain sections showing the rostral to caudal extent of the striatum, the region of interest in which DAT, VMAT2, D$_1$, D$_2$, and D$_3$ receptors were quantified, across a total of six sections (g). NSB, nonspecific binding; Str, striatum. *$p < 0.05$ for *Pink1* knockout rat vs. control rat.

Figure 9 (Howes et al., 2013)

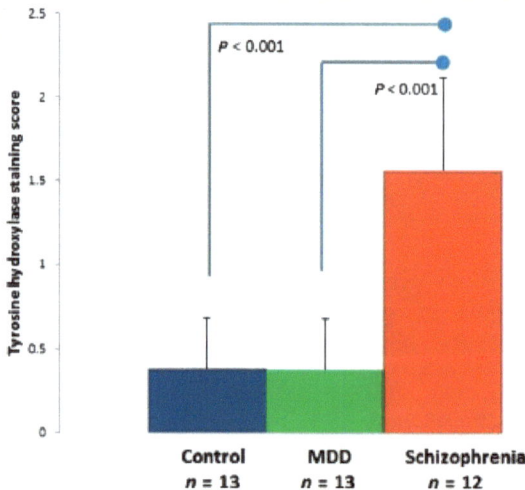

Figure 1 Median (IQR) staining scores for tyrosine hydroxylase levels in substantia nigra for control subjects ($n = 13$); major depressive disorder (MDD, $n = 13$); and schizophrenia ($n = 12$).

Figure 10 (Seeman and Tinazzi, 2013)

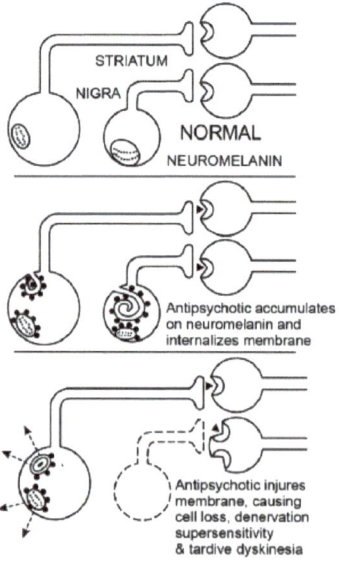

Fig. 3. Long-term use of antipsychotics leads to drug accumulation (Seeman, 1988) in the neuromelanin of the dopamine-containing neurons in the substantia nigra (top and middle panels), with internalization of the cell membranes (Jellinger, 1977; Tousimis and Barron, 1970) (middle panel), and subsequent injury to the cell membranes (bottom panel), leading to dopamine supersensitivity and tardive dyskinesia. Adapted and redrawn from Seeman (1988).

References

Albin, R. L., Young, A. B., & Penney, J. B. (1989). The functional anatomy of basal ganglia disorders. *Trends Neurosci, 12*(10), 366-375

Alexander, G. E., Crutcher, M. D., & DeLong, M. R. (1990). Basal ganglia-thalamocortical circuits: parallel substrates for motor, oculomotor, "prefrontal" and "limbic" functions. *Prog Brain Res, 85*, 119-146

Arias-Carrion, O., Stamelou, M., Murillo-Rodriguez, E., Menendez-Gonzalez, M., & Poppel, E. (2010). Dopaminergic reward system: a short integrative review. *International Archives of Medicine, 3*, 1-6. doi: 10.1186/1755-7682-3-24

Beaudry, G., Langlois, M. C., Weppe, I., Rouillard, C., & Levesque, D. (2000). Contrasting patterns and cellular specificity of transcriptional regulation of the nuclear receptor nerve growth factor-inducible B by haloperidol and clozapine in the rat forebrain. *J Neurochem, 75*(4), 1694-1702

Bertran-Gonzalez, J., Bosch, C., Maroteaux, M., Matamales, M., Herve, D., Valjent, E., & Girault, J. A. (2008). Opposing patterns of signaling activation in dopamine D1 and D2 receptor-expressing striatal neurons in response to cocaine and haloperidol. *J Neurosci, 28*(22), 5671-5685. doi: 10.1523/jneurosci.1039-08.2008

Birrell, J. M., & Brown, V. J. (2000). Medial frontal cortex mediates perceptual attentional set shifting in the rat. *J Neurosci, 20*(11), 4320-4324

Bjorklund, A., & Dunnett, S. B. (2007). Dopamine neuron systems in the brain: an update. *Trends Neurosci, 30*(5), 194-202. doi: 10.1016/j.tins.2007.03.006

Bolam, J. P., Hanley, J. J., Booth, P. A., & Bevan, M. D. (2000). Synaptic organization of the basal ganglia. *J Anat, 196 (Pt 4)*, 527-542

Bologna, M., Conte, A., Suppa, A., & Berardelli, A. (2012). Motor cortex plasticity in Parkinson's disease: advances and controversies. *Clinical Neurophysiology, 123*(4), 640-641. doi: 10.1016/j.clinph.2011.08.021

Borodinsky, L. N., Belgacem, Y. H., Swapna, I., & Sequerra, E. B. (2014). Dynamic regulation of neurotransmitter specification: relevance to nervous system homeostasis. *Neuropharmacology, 78*, 75-80. doi: 10.1016/j.neuropharm.2012.12.005

Britt, J. P., Benaliouad, F., McDevitt, R. A., Stuber, G. D., Wise, R. A., & Bonci, A. (2012). Synaptic and behavioral profile of multiple glutamatergic inputs to the nucleus accumbens. *Neuron, 76*(4), 790-803. doi: 10.1016/j.neuron.2012.09.040

Britt, J. P., & Bonci, A. (2013). Optogenetic interrogations of the neural circuits underlying addiction. *Current Opinion in Neurobiology, 23*(4), 539-545. doi: 10.1016/j.conb.2013.01.010

Brooks, A. M., & Berns, G. S. (2013). Aversive stimuli and loss in the mesocorticolimbic dopamine system. *Trends in Cognitive Sciences, 17*(6), 281-286. doi: 10.1016/j.tics.2013.04.001

Carli, M., Evenden, J. L., & Robbins, T. W. (1985). Depletion of unilateral striatal dopamine impairs initiation of contralateral actions and not sensory attention. *Nature, 313*(6004), 679-682

Carli, M., Jones, G. H., & Robbins, T. W. (1989). Effects of unilateral dorsal and ventral striatal dopamine depletion on visual neglect in the rat: a neural and behavioral analysis. *Neuroscience, 29*(2), 309-327

Carlsson, A. (1974). Antipsychotic drugs and catecholamine synapses. *J Psychiatr Res, 11*, 57-64

Carlsson, A. (1978). Antipsychotic drugs, neurotransmitters, and schizophrenia. *Am J Psychiatry, 135*(2), 165-173

Carlsson, A. (2002). Treatment of Parkinson's with L-DOPA. The early discovery phase, and a comment on current problems. *J Neural Transm, 109*(5-6), 777-787. doi: 10.1007/s007020200064

Castillo, S. O., Baffi, J. S., Palkovits, M., Goldstein, D. S., Kopin, I. J., Witta, J., . . . Nikodem, V. M. (1998). Dopamine biosynthesis is selectively abolished in substantia nigra/ventral tegmental area but not in hypothalamic neurons in mice with targeted disruption of the Nurr1 gene. *Mol Cell Neurosci, 11*(1-2), 36-46. doi: 10.1006/mcne.1998.0673

Castrioto, A., Lhommee, E., Moro, E., & Krack, P. (2014). Mood and behavioral effects of subthalamic stimulation in Parkinson's disease. *Lancet Neurology, 13*(3), 287-305. doi: 10.1016/s1474-4422(13)70294-1

Cazorla, P., Smidt, M. P., O'Malley, K. L., & Burbach, J. P. (2000). A response element for the homeodomain transcription factor Ptx3 in the tyrosine hydroxylase gene promoter. *J Neurochem, 74*(5), 1829-1837

Cha, D. S., Kudlow, P. A., Baskaran, A., Mansur, R. B., & McIntyre, R. S. (2014). Implications of epigenetic modulation for novel treatment approaches in patients with schizophrenia. *Neuropharmacology, 77*, 481-486. doi: 10.1016/j.neuropharm.2013.08.038

Choi, Y. M., Jang, J. Y., Jang, M., Kim, S. H., Kang, Y. K., Cho, H., . . . Park, M. K. (2009). Modulation of firing activity by ATP in dopamine neurons of the rat substantia nigra pars compacta. *Neuroscience, 160*(3), 587-595. doi: 10.1016/j.neuroscience.2009.02.067

Chudasama, Y., & Robbins, T. W. (2003). Dissociable contributions of the orbitofrontal and infralimbic cortex to pavlovian autoshaping and discrimination reversal learning: further evidence for the functional heterogeneity of the rodent frontal cortex. *J Neurosci, 23*(25), 8771-8780

Consortium, C.-D. G. o. t. P. G., & Consortium, G. R. O. o. P. G. (2013). Identification of risk loci with shared effects on five major psychiatric disorders: a genome-wide analysis. *Lancet, 381*(9875), 1371-1379. doi: 10.1016/s0140-6736(12)62129-1

Coppede, F. (2012). Genetics and epigenetics of Parkinson's disease. *The Scientific World Journal, 2012*, 1-12. doi: 10.1100/2012/489830

Crow, T. J. (1973). Catecholamine-containing neurons and electrical self-stimulation. 2. A theoretical interpretation and some psychiatric implications. *Psychol Med, 3*(1), 66-73

da Silva Lobo, D. S., Vallada, H. P., Knight, J., Martins, S. S., Tavares, H., Gentil, V., & Kennedy, J. L. (2007). Dopamine genes and pathological gambling in discordant sib-pairs. *J Gambl Stud, 23*(4), 421-433. doi: 10.1007/s10899-007-9060-x

Daubner, S. C., Lauriano, C., Haycock, J. W., & Fitzpatrick, P. F. (1992). Site-directed mutagenesis of serine 40 of rat tyrosine hydroxylase. Effects of dopamine and cAMP-dependent phosphorylation on enzyme activity. *J Biol Chem, 267*(18), 12639-12646

Davis, K. L., Kahn, R. S., Ko, G., & Davidson, M. (1991). Dopamine in schizophrenia: a review and reconceptualization. *Am J Psychiatry, 148*(11), 1474-1486

De Bellis, M. D. (2002). Developmental traumatology: a contributory mechanism for alcohol and substance use disorders. *Psychoneuroendocrinology, 27*(1-2), 155-170

DeLong, M. R., & Wichmann, T. (2007). Circuits and circuit disorders of the basal ganglia. *Arch Neurol, 64*(1), 20-24. doi: 10.1001/archneur.64.1.20

Demjaha, A., Murray, R. M., McGuire, P. K., Kapur, S., & Howes, O. D. (2012). Dopamine synthesis capacity in patients with treatment-resistant schizophrenia. *Am J Psychiatry, 169*(11), 1203-1210. doi: 10.1176/appi.ajp.2012.12010144

Dexter, D. T., & Jenner, P. (2013). Parkinson disease: from pathology to molecular disease mechanisms. *Free Radical Biology & Medicine, 62*, 132-144. doi: 10.1016/j.freeradbiomed.2013.01.018

Di Chiara, G., & Imperato, A. (1988). Drugs abused by humans preferentially increase synaptic dopamine concentrations in the mesolimbic system of freely moving rats. *Proc Natl Acad Sci U S A, 85*(14), 5274-5278

Dunah, A. W., Wang, Y., Yasuda, R. P., Kameyama, K., Huganir, R. L., Wolfe, B. B., & Standaert, D. G. (2000). Alterations in subunit expression, composition, and phosphorylation of striatal N-methyl-D-aspartate glutamate receptors in a rat 6-hydroxydopamine model of Parkinson's disease. *Mol Pharmacol, 57*(2), 342-352

Eagle, D. M., Baunez, C., Hutcheson, D. M., Lehmann, O., Shah, A. P., & Robbins, T. W. (2008). Stop-signal reaction-time task performance: role of prefrontal cortex and subthalamic nucleus. *Cereb Cortex, 18*(1), 178-188. doi: 10.1093/cercor/bhm044

Eells, J. B., Lipska, B. K., Yeung, S. K., Misler, J. A., & Nikodem, V. M. (2002). Nurr1-null heterozygous mice have reduced mesolimbic and mesocortical dopamine levels and increased stress-induced locomotor activity. *Behav Brain Res, 136*(1), 267-275

Ethier, I., Beaudry, G., St-Hilaire, M., Milbrandt, J., Rouillard, C., & Levesque, D. (2004). The transcription factor NGFI-B (Nur77) and retinoids play a critical role in acute neuroleptic-induced extrapyramidal effect and striatal neuropeptide gene expression. *Neuropsychopharmacology, 29*(2), 335-346. doi: 10.1038/sj.npp.1300318

Fariello, R. G., & Hornykiewicz, O. (1979). Substantia nigra and pentylenetetrazol threshold in rats: correlation with striatal dopamine metabolism. *Exp Neurol, 65*(1), 202-208

Fields, H. L., Hjelmstad, G. O., Margolis, E. B., & Nicola, S. M. (2007). Ventral tegmental area neurons in learned appetitive behavior and positive reinforcement. *Annu Rev Neurosci, 30*, 289-316. doi: 10.1146/annurev.neuro.30.051606.094341

Fischle, W., Dequiedt, F., Hendzel, M. J., Guenther, M. G., Lazar, M. A., Voelter, W., & Verdin, E. (2002). Enzymatic activity associated with class II HDACs is dependent on a multiprotein complex containing HDAC3 and SMRT/N-CoR. *Mol Cell, 9*(1), 45-57

Floresco, S. B., St Onge, J. R., Ghods-Sharifi, S., & Winstanley, C. A. (2008). Cortico-limbic-striatal circuits subserving different forms of cost-benefit decision making. *Cogn Affect Behav Neurosci, 8*(4), 375-389. doi: 10.3758/cabn.8.4.375

Floresco, S. B., Zhang, Y., & Enomoto, T. (2009). Neural circuits subserving behavioral flexibility and their relevance to schizophrenia. *Behav Brain Res, 204*(2), 396-409. doi: 10.1016/j.bbr.2008.12.001

Gerfen, C. R. (1984). The neostriatal mosaic: compartmentalization of corticostriatal input and striatonigral output systems. *Nature, 311*(5985), 461-464

Gerfen, C. R. (1992). The neostriatal mosaic: multiple levels of compartmental organization. *Trends*

German, D. C., & Manaye, K. F. (1993). Midbrain dopaminergic neurons (nuclei A8, A9, and A10): three-dimensional reconstruction in the rat. *J Comp Neurol, 331*(3), 297-309. doi: 10.1002/cne.903310302

Goldberg, J. H., Farries, M. A., & Fee, M. S. (2013). Basal ganglia output to the thalamus: still a paradox. *Trends Neurosci, 36*(12), 695-705. doi: 10.1016/j.tins.2013.09.001

Goldstein, R. Z., & Volkow, N. D. (2002). Drug addiction and its underlying neurobiological basis: neuroimaging evidence for the involvement of the frontal cortex. *The American Journal of Psychiatry, 159*(10), 1642-1652

Gong, S., Zheng, C., Doughty, M. L., Losos, K., Didkovsky, N., Schambra, U. B., . . . Heintz, N. (2003). A gene expression atlas of the central nervous system based on bacterial artificial chromosomes. *Nature, 425*(6961), 917-925. doi: 10.1038/nature02033

Guatteo, E., Yee, A., McKearney, J., Cucchiaroni, M. L., Armogida, M., Berretta, N., . . . Lipski, J. (2013). Dual effects of L-DOPA on nigral dopaminergic neurons. *Experimental Neurology, 247*, 582-594. doi: 10.1016/j.expneurol.2013.02.009

Guenther, M. G., Barak, O., & Lazar, M. A. (2001). The SMRT and N-CoR corepressors are activating cofactors for histone deacetylase 3. *Mol Cell Biol, 21*(18), 6091-6101

Haavik, J., & Toska, K. (1998). Tyrosine hydroxylase and Parkinson's disease. *Mol Neurobiol, 16*(3), 285-309. doi: 10.1007/bf02741387

Haber, S. N. (2003). The primate basal ganglia: parallel and integrative networks. *J Chem Neuroanat, 26*(4), 317-330

He, Y., Yu, S., Bae, E., Shen, H., & Wang, Y. (2013). Methamphetamine alters reference gene expression in nigra and striatum of adult rat brain. *Neurotoxicology, 39*, 138-145. doi: 10.1016/j.neuro.2013.08.009

Holt, D. J., Graybiel, A. M., & Saper, C. B. (1997). Neurochemical architecture of the human striatum. *J Comp Neurol, 384*(1), 1-25

Horn, A. S., & Snyder, S. H. (1971). Chlorpromazine and dopamine: conformational similarities that correlate with the antischizophrenic activity of phenothiazine drugs. *Proc Natl Acad Sci U S A, 68*(10), 2325-2328

Howell, L. L., & Kimmel, H. L. (2008). Monoamine transporters and psychostimulant addiction. *Biochemical Pharmacology, 75*(1), 196-217. doi: 10.1016/j.bcp.2007.08.003

Howes, O. D., Egerton, A., Allan, V., McGuire, P., Stokes, P., & Kapur, S. (2009). Mechanisms underlying psychosis and antipsychotic treatment response in schizophrenia: insights from PET and SPECT imaging. *Curr Pharm Des, 15*(22), 2550-2559

Howes, O. D., & Kapur, S. (2009). The dopamine hypothesis of schizophrenia: version III--the final common pathway. *Schizophr Bull, 35*(3), 549-562. doi: 10.1093/schbul/sbp006

Howes, O. D., Montgomery, A. J., Asselin, M. C., Murray, R. M., Grasby, P. M., & McGuire, P. K. (2007). Molecular imaging studies of the striatal dopaminergic system in psychosis and predictions for the prodromal phase of psychosis. *Br J Psychiatry Suppl, 51*, s13-18. doi: 10.1192/bjp.191.51.s13

Howes, O. D., Williams, M., Ibrahim, K., Leung, G., Egerton, A., McGuire, P. K., & Turkheimer, F. (2013). Midbrain dopamine function in schizophrenia and depression: a post-mortem and positron emission tomographic imaging study. *Brain, 136*(Pt 11), 3242-3251. doi: 10.1093/brain/awt264

Huang, E. Y., Zhang, J., Miska, E. A., Guenther, M. G., Kouzarides, T., & Lazar, M. A. (2000). Nuclear receptor corepressors partner with class II histone deacetylases in a Sin3-independent repression pathway. *Genes Dev, 14*(1), 45-54

Iacovelli, L., Fulceri, F., De Blasi, A., Nicoletti, F., Ruggieri, S., & Fornai, F. (2006). The neurotoxicity of amphetamines: bridging drugs of abuse and neurodegenerative disorders. *Experimental Neurology, 201*(1), 24-31. doi: 10.1016/j.expneurol.2006.02.130

Ikemoto, S., & Bonci, A. (2014). Neurocircuitry of drug reward. *Neuropharmacology, 76 B*, 329-341. doi: 10.1016/j.neuropharm.2013.04.031

Jacobs, F. M., van der Linden, A. J., Wang, Y., von Oerthel, L., Sul, H. S., Burbach, J. P., & Smidt, M. P. (2009). Identification of Dlk1, Ptpru and Klhl1 as novel Nurr1 target genes in mesodiencephalic dopamine neurons. *Development, 136*(14), 2363-2373. doi: 10.1242/dev.037556

Jacobs, F. M., van der Linden, A. J., Wang, Y., von Oerthel, L., Sul, H. S., Burbach, J. P., & Smidt, M. P. (2009). Identification of Dlk1, Ptpru and Klhl1 as novel Nurr1 target genes in mesodiencephalic dopamine neurons. *Development, 136*(14), 2363-2373. doi: 10.1242/dev.037556

Jacobs, F. M., van Erp, S., van der Linden, A. J., von Oerthel, L., Burbach, J. P., & Smidt, M. P. (2009). Pitx3 potentiates Nurr1 in dopamine neuron terminal differentiation through release of SMRT-mediated repression. *Development, 136*(4), 531-540. doi: 10.1242/dev.029769

Jang, M., Jang, J. Y., Kim, S. H., Uhm, K. B., Kang, Y. K., Kim, H. J., . . . Park, M. K. (2011). Functional organization of dendritic Ca2+ signals in midbrain dopamine neurons. *Cell Calcium, 50*(4), 370-380. doi: 10.1016/j.ceca.2011.06.007

Jankovic, J., Chen, S., & Le, W. D. (2005). The role of Nurr1 in the development of dopaminergic neurons and Parkinson's disease. *Prog Neurobiol, 77*(1-2), 128-138. doi: 10.1016/j.pneurobio.2005.09.001

Jankovic, J., Chen, S., & Le, W. D. (2005). The role of Nurr1 in the development of dopaminergic neurons and Parkinson's disease. *Prog Neurobiol, 77*(1-2), 128-138. doi: 10.1016/j.pneurobio.2005.09.001

Jenner, P. (2008). Molecular mechanisms of L-DOPA-induced dyskinesia. *Nature Reviews. Neuroscience, 9*(9), 665-677. doi: 10.1038/nrn2471

Jog, M. S., Kubota, Y., Connolly, C. I., Hillegaart, V., & Graybiel, A. M. (1999). Building neural representations of habits. *Science, 286*(5445), 1745-1749

Kadkhodaei, B., Ito, T., Joodmardi, E., Mattsson, B., Rouillard, C., Carta, M., . . . Perlmann, T. (2009). Nurr1 is required for maintenance of maturing and adult midbrain dopamine neurons. *J Neurosci, 29*(50), 15923-15932. doi: 10.1523/jneurosci.3910-09.2009

Kawaguchi, Y. (1997). Neostriatal cell subtypes and their functional roles. *Neurosci Res, 27*(1), 1-8

Kelley, A. E., & Berridge, K. C. (2002). The neuroscience of natural rewards: relevance to addictive drugs. *J Neurosci, 22*(9), 3306-3311. doi: 20026361

Kim, K. S., Kim, C. H., Hwang, D. Y., Seo, H., Chung, S., Hong, S. J., . . . Isacson, O. (2003). Orphan nuclear receptor Nurr1 directly transactivates the promoter activity of the tyrosine hydroxylase gene in a cell-specific manner. *J Neurochem, 85*(3), 622-634

Kim, S. H., Jang, J. Y., Jang, M., Um, K. B., Chung, S., Kim, H. J., & Park, M. K. (2013).

Homeostatic regulation mechanism of spontaneous firing determines glutamate responsiveness in the midbrain dopamine neurons. *Cell Calcium, 54*(4), 295-306. doi: 10.1016/j.ceca.2013.07.004

Koob, G. F., & Volkow, N. D. (2010). Neurocircuitry of addiction. *Neuropsychopharmacology, 35*(1), 217-238. doi: 10.1038/npp.2009.110

Koob, G. F., & Weiss, F. (1992). Neuropharmacology of cocaine and ethanol dependence. *Recent Dev Alcohol, 10*, 201-233

Korchounov, A., Meyer, M. F., & Krasnianski, M. (2010). Postsynaptic nigrostriatal dopamine receptors and their role in movement regulation. *Journal of Neural Transmission, 117*(12), 1359-1369. doi: 10.1007/s00702-010-0454-z

Krasnova, I. N., Chiflikyan, M., Justinova, Z., McCoy, M. T., Ladenheim, B., Jayanthi, S., . . . Cadet, J. L. (2013). CREB phosphorylation regulates striatal transcriptional responses in the self-administration model of methamphetamine addiction in the rat. *Neurobiology of Disease, 58*, 132-143. doi: 10.1016/j.nbd.2013.05.009

Kravitz, A. V., Owen, S. F., & Kreitzer, A. C. (2013). Optogenetic identification of striatal projection neuron subtypes during in vivo recordings. *Brain Research, 1511*, 21-32. doi: 10.1016/j.brainres.2012.11.018

Lammel, S., Ion, D. I., Roeper, J., & Malenka, R. C. (2011). Projection-specific modulation of dopamine neuron synapses by aversive and rewarding stimuli. *Neuron, 70*(5), 855-862. doi: 10.1016/j.neuron.2011.03.025

Lammel, S., Lim, B. K., & Malenka, R. C. (2014). Reward and aversion in a heterogeneous midbrain dopamine system. *Neuropharmacology, 76 B*, 351-359. doi: 10.1016/j.neuropharm.2013.03.019

Le Moal, M., & Simon, H. (1991). Mesocorticolimbic dopaminergic network: functional and regulatory roles. *Physiol Rev, 71*(1), 155-234

Le, W., Pan, T., Huang, M., Xu, P., Xie, W., Zhu, W., . . . Jankovic, J. (2008). Decreased NURR1 gene expression in patients with Parkinson's disease. *J Neurol Sci, 273*(1-2), 29-33. doi: 10.1016/j.jns.2008.06.007

Lee, S. P., So, C. H., Rashid, A. J., Varghese, G., Cheng, R., Lanca, A. J., . . . George, S. R. (2004). Dopamine D1 and D2 receptor Co-activation generates a novel phospholipase C-mediated calcium signal. *J Biol Chem, 279*(34), 35671-35678. doi: 10.1074/jbc.M401923200

Lenz, J. D., & Lobo, M. K. (2013). Optogenetic insights into striatal function and behavior. *Behavioural Brain Research, 255*, 44-54. doi: 10.1016/j.bbr.2013.04.018

Levine, M. S., Li, Z., Cepeda, C., Cromwell, H. C., & Altemus, K. L. (1996). Neuromodulatory actions of dopamine on synaptically-evoked neostriatal responses in slices. *Synapse, 24*(1), 65-78. doi: 10.1002/syn.890240102

Lohmann, E., Thobois, S., Lesage, S., Broussolle, E., du Montcel, S. T., Ribeiro, M. J., . . . Brice, A. (2009). A multidisciplinary study of patients with early-onset PD with and without parkin mutations. *Neurology, 72*(2), 110-116. doi: 10.1212/01.wnl.0000327098.86861.d4

London, E. D., Morgan, M. J., Phillips, R. L., Stapleton, J. M., Cascella, N. G., & Wong, D. F. (1990). Mapping the metabolic correlates of drug-induced euphoria. *NIDA Res Monogr, 105*, 54-60

Luscher, C., & Malenka, R. C. (2011). Drug-evoked synaptic plasticity in addiction: from molecular changes to circuit remodeling. *Neuron, 69*(4), 650-663. doi: 10.1016/j.neuron.2011.01.017

Lyon, G. J., Abi-Dargham, A., Moore, H., Lieberman, J. A., Javitch, J. A., & Sulzer, D. (2011). Presynaptic regulation of dopamine transmission in schizophrenia. *Schizophr Bull, 37*(1), 108-117. doi: 10.1093/schbul/sbp010

Lyon, G. J., Abi-Dargham, A., Moore, H., Lieberman, J. A., Javitch, J. A., & Sulzer, D. (2011). Presynaptic regulation of dopamine transmission in schizophrenia. *Schizophr Bull, 37*(1), 108-117. doi: 10.1093/schbul/sbp010

Maddux, J. M., & Holland, P. C. (2011). Dissociations between medial prefrontal cortical subregions in the modulation of learning and action. *Behav Neurosci, 125*(3), 383-395. doi: 10.1037/a0023515

Mahmoudi, S., Samadi, P., Gilbert, F., Ouattara, B., Morissette, M., Gregoire, L., . . . Levesque, D. (2009). Nur77 mRNA levels and L-Dopa-induced dyskinesias in MPTP monkeys treated with docosahexaenoic acid. *Neurobiol Dis, 36*(1), 213-222. doi: 10.1016/j.nbd.2009.07.017

Malvaez, M., Mhillaj, E., Matheos, D. P., Palmery, M., & Wood, M. A. (2011). CBP in the nucleus accumbens regulates cocaine-induced histone acetylation and is critical for cocaine-associated behaviors. *J Neurosci, 31*(47), 16941-16948. doi: 10.1523/jneurosci.2747-11.2011

Martinat, C., Bacci, J. J., Leete, T., Kim, J., Vanti, W. B., Newman, A. H., . . . Abeliovich, A. (2006). Cooperative transcription activation by Nurr1 and Pitx3 induces embryonic stem cell maturation to the midbrain dopamine neuron phenotype. *Proc Natl Acad Sci U S A, 103*(8), 2874-2879. doi: 10.1073/pnas.0511153103

Maze, I., Covington, H. E., 3rd, Dietz, D. M., LaPlant, Q., Renthal, W., Russo, S. J., . . . Nestler, E. J. (2010). Essential role of the histone methyltransferase G9a in cocaine-induced plasticity. *Science, 327*(5962), 213-216. doi: 10.1126/science.1179438

McAlonan, K., & Brown, V. J. (2003). Orbital prefrontal cortex mediates reversal learning and not attentional set shifting in the rat. *Behav Brain Res, 146*(1-2), 97-103

McCulloch, R. I., Daubner, S. C., & Fitzpatrick, P. F. (2001). Effects of substitution at serine 40 of tyrosine hydroxylase on catecholamine binding. *Biochemistry, 40*(24), 7273-7278

Meisenzahl, E. M., Schmitt, G. J., Scheuerecker, J., & Moller, H. J. (2007). The role of dopamine for the pathophysiology of schizophrenia. *Int Rev Psychiatry, 19*(4), 337-345. doi: 10.1080/09540260701502468

Meisenzahl, E. M., Schmitt, G. J., Scheuerecker, J., & Moller, H. J. (2007). The role of dopamine for the pathophysiology of schizophrenia. *Int Rev Psychiatry, 19*(4), 337-345. doi: 10.1080/09540260701502468

Meltzer, H. Y., & Stahl, S. M. (1976). The dopamine hypothesis of schizophrenia: a review. *Schizophr Bull, 2*(1), 19-76

Missale, C., Nash, S. R., Robinson, S. W., Jaber, M., & Caron, M. G. (1998). Dopamine receptors: from structure to function. *Physiol Rev, 78*(1), 189-225

Muly, E. C., 3rd, Szigeti, K., & Goldman-Rakic, P. S. (1998). D1 receptor in interneurons of macaque prefrontal cortex: distribution and subcellular localization. *J Neurosci, 18*(24), 10553-10565

Muschamp, J. W., & Carlezon, W. A., Jr. (2013). Roles of nucleus accumbens CREB and dynorphin in dysregulation of motivation. *Cold Spring Harb Perspect Med, 3*(2), a012005. doi: 10.1101/cshperspect.a012005

Nesse, R. M., & Berridge, K. C. (1997). Psychoactive drug use in evolutionary perspective. *Science,*

278(5335), 63-66

Nestler, E. J. (2005). The neurobiology of cocaine addiction. *Sci Pract Perspect, 3*(1), 4-10

Nestler, E. J. (2014). Epigenetic mechanisms of drug addiction. *Neuropharmacology, 76 B*, 259-268. doi: 10.1016/j.neuropharm.2013.04.004

Nicola, S. M. (2007). The nucleus accumbens as part of a basal ganglia action selection circuit. *Psychopharmacology (Berl), 191*(3), 521-550. doi: 10.1007/s00213-006-0510-4

Nieh, E. H., Kim, S. Y., Namburi, P., & Tye, K. M. (2013). Optogenetic dissection of neural circuits underlying emotional valence and motivated behaviors. *Brain Research, 1511*, 73-92. doi: 10.1016/j.brainres.2012.11.001

Olds, J., & Milner, P. (1954). Positive reinforcement produced by electrical stimulation of septal area and other regions of rat brain. *J Comp Physiol Psychol, 47*(6), 419-427

Panksepp, J., Knutson, B., & Burgdorf, J. (2002). The role of brain emotional systems in addictions: a neuro-evolutionary perspective and new 'self-report' animal model. *Addiction, 97*(4), 459-469

Peled, A. (2011). Optogenetic neuronal control in schizophrenia. *Medical Hypotheses, 76*(6), 914-921. doi: 10.1016/j.mehy.2011.03.009

Phan, K. L., Wager, T., Taylor, S. F., & Liberzon, I. (2002). Functional neuroanatomy of emotion: a meta-analysis of emotion activation studies in PET and fMRI. *Neuroimage, 16*(2), 331-348. doi: 10.1006/nimg.2002.1087

Pierce, R. C., & Kalivas, P. W. (1997). A circuitry model of the expression of behavioral sensitization to amphetamine-like psychostimulants. *Brain Res Brain Res Rev, 25*(2), 192-216

Robison, A. J., & Nestler, E. J. (2011). Transcriptional and epigenetic mechanisms of addiction. *Nat Rev Neurosci, 12*(11), 623-637. doi: 10.1038/nrn3111

Rojas, P., Ruiz-Sanchez, E., Rojas, C., & Ogren, S. O. (2012). Ginkgo biloba extract (EGb 761) modulates the expression of dopamine-related genes in 1-methyl-4-phenyl-1,2,3,6-tetrahydropyridine-induced Parkinsonism in mice. *Neuroscience, 223*, 246-257. doi: 10.1016/j.neuroscience.2012.08.004

Rondou, P., Haegeman, G., & Van Craenenbroeck, K. (2010). The dopamine D4 receptor: biochemical and signaling properties. *Cell Mol Life Sci, 67*(12), 1971-1986. doi: 10.1007/s00018-010-0293-y

Rousseaux, M. W., Marcogliese, P. C., Qu, D., Hewitt, S. J., Seang, S., Kim, R. H., . . . Park, D. S. (2012). Progressive dopaminergic cell loss with unilateral-to-bilateral progression in a genetic model of Parkinson disease. *Proc Natl Acad Sci U S A, 109*(39), 15918-15923. doi: 10.1073/pnas.1205102109

Russo, S. J., Dietz, D. M., Dumitriu, D., Morrison, J. H., Malenka, R. C., & Nestler, E. J. (2010). Addicted synapse: mechanisms of synaptic and structural plasticity in nucleus accumbens. *Trends in Neurosciences, 33*(6), 267-276. doi: 10.1016/j.tins.2010.02.002

Sakurada, K., Ohshima-Sakurada, M., Palmer, T. D., & Gage, F. H. (1999). Nurr1, an orphan nuclear receptor, is a transcriptional activator of endogenous tyrosine hydroxylase in neural progenitor cells derived from the adult brain. *Development, 126*(18), 4017-4026

Salamone, J. D., Correa, M., Farrar, A., & Mingote, S. M. (2007). Effort-related functions of nucleus accumbens dopamine and associated forebrain circuits. *Psychopharmacology (Berl), 191*(3), 461-482.

doi: 10.1007/s00213-006-0668-9

Salvatore, M. F., & Pruett, B. S. (2012). Dichotomy of tyrosine hydroxylase and dopamine regulation between somatodendritic and terminal field areas of nigrostriatal and mesoaccumbens pathways. *PLoS One, 7*(1), e29867. doi: 10.1371/journal.pone.0029867

Sanchez, N., Coura, R., Engmann, O., Marion-Poll, L., Longueville, S., Herve, D., . . . Girault, J. A. (2014). Haloperidol-induced Nur77 expression in striatopallidal neurons is under the control of protein phosphatase 1 regulation by DARPP-32. *Neuropharmacology, 79*, 559-566. doi: 10.1016/j.neuropharm.2014.01.008

Saucedo-Cardenas, O., Quintana-Hau, J. D., Le, W. D., Smidt, M. P., Cox, J. J., De Mayo, F., . . . Conneely, O. M. (1998). Nurr1 is essential for the induction of the dopaminergic phenotype and the survival of ventral mesencephalic late dopaminergic precursor neurons. *Proc Natl Acad Sci U S A, 95*(7), 4013-4018

Seeman, P. (2006). Targeting the dopamine D2 receptor in schizophrenia. *Expert Opin Ther Targets, 10*(4), 515-531. doi: 10.1517/14728222.10.4.515

Seeman, P., Chau-Wong, M., Tedesco, J., & Wong, K. (1975). Brain receptors for antipsychotic drugs and dopamine: direct binding assays. *Proc Natl Acad Sci U S A, 72*(11), 4376-4380

Sesack, S. R., Snyder, C. L., & Lewis, D. A. (1995). Axon terminals immunolabeled for dopamine or tyrosine hydroxylase synapse on GABA-immunoreactive dendrites in rat and monkey cortex. *J Comp Neurol, 363*(2), 264-280. doi: 10.1002/cne.903630208

Shotbolt, P., Stokes, P. R., Owens, S. F., Toulopoulou, T., Picchioni, M. M., Bose, S. K., . . . Howes, O. D. (2011). Striatal dopamine synthesis capacity in twins discordant for schizophrenia. *Psychol Med, 41*(11), 2331-2338. doi: 10.1017/s0033291711000341

Sibley, D. R., Monsma, F. J., Jr., McVittie, L. D., Gerfen, C. R., Burch, R. M., & Mahan, L. C. (1992). Molecular neurobiology of dopamine receptor subtypes. *Neurochem Int, 20 Suppl*, 17s-22s

Sikazwe, D. M., Li, S., Mardenborough, L., Cody, V., Roth, B. L., & Ablordeppey, S. Y. (2004). Haloperidol: towards further understanding of the structural contributions of its pharmacophoric elements at D2-like receptors. *Bioorg Med Chem Lett, 14*(23), 5739-5742. doi: 10.1016/j.bmcl.2004.09.046

Sklair-Tavron, L., Shi, W. X., Lane, S. B., Harris, H. W., Bunney, B. S., & Nestler, E. J. (1996). Chronic morphine induces visible changes in the morphology of mesolimbic dopamine neurons. *Proc Natl Acad Sci U S A, 93*(20), 11202-11207

Snyder, S. H. (1972). Catecholamines in the brain as mediators of amphetamine psychosis. *Arch Gen Psychiatry, 27*(2), 169-179

Steiner, H., & Gerfen, C. R. (1999). Enkephalin regulates acute D2 dopamine receptor antagonist-induced immediate-early gene expression in striatal neurons. *Neuroscience, 88*(3), 795-810

Sun, J., Kouranova, E., Cui, X., Mach, R. H., & Xu, J. (2013). Regulation of dopamine presynaptic markers and receptors in the striatum of DJ-1 and Pink1 knockout rats. *Neurosci Lett, 557 Pt B*, 123-128. doi: 10.1016/j.neulet.2013.10.034

Sun, L., Li, Q., Li, Q., Zhang, Y., Liu, D., Jiang, H., . . . Yew, D. T. (2014). Chronic ketamine exposure induces permanent impairment of brain functions in adolescent cynomolgus monkeys. *Addict Biol, 19*(2), 185-194. doi: 10.1111/adb.12004

Sura, G. R., Daubner, S. C., & Fitzpatrick, P. F. (2004). Effects of phosphorylation by protein kinase A on binding of catecholamines to the human tyrosine hydroxylase isoforms. *J Neurochem, 90*(4), 970-978. doi: 10.1111/j.1471-4159.2004.02566.x

Sutherland, C., Alterio, J., Campbell, D. G., Le Bourdelles, B., Mallet, J., Haavik, J., & Cohen, P. (1993). Phosphorylation and activation of human tyrosine hydroxylase in vitro by mitogen-activated protein (MAP) kinase and MAP-kinase-activated kinases 1 and 2. *Eur J Biochem, 217*(2), 715-722

Swanson, L. W. (1982). The projections of the ventral tegmental area and adjacent regions: a combined fluorescent retrograde tracer and immunofluorescence study in the rat. *Brain Res Bull, 9*(1-6), 321-353

Thanos, P. K., Michaelides, M., Benveniste, H., Wang, G. J., & Volkow, N. D. (2007). Effects of chronic oral methylphenidate on cocaine self-administration and striatal dopamine D2 receptors in rodents. *Pharmacol Biochem Behav, 87*(4), 426-433. doi: 10.1016/j.pbb.2007.05.020

Thanos, P. K., Volkow, N. D., Freimuth, P., Umegaki, H., Ikari, H., Roth, G., . . . Hitzemann, R. (2001). Overexpression of dopamine D2 receptors reduces alcohol self-administration. *J Neurochem, 78*(5), 1094-1103

Tinazzi, M., Cipriani, A., Matinella, A., Cannas, A., Solla, P., Nicoletti, A., . . . Barbui, C. (2012). [(1)(2)(3)I]FP-CIT single photon emission computed tomography findings in drug-induced Parkinsonism. *Schizophr Res, 139*(1-3), 40-45. doi: 10.1016/j.schres.2012.06.003

Tsankova, N., Renthal, W., Kumar, A., & Nestler, E. J. (2007). Epigenetic regulation in psychiatric disorders. *Nat Rev Neurosci, 8*(5), 355-367. doi: 10.1038/nrn2132

Tseng, K. Y., Roubert, C., Do, L., Rubinstein, M., Kelly, M. A., Grandy, D. K., . . . Raisman-Vozari, R. (2000). Selective increase of Nurr1 mRNA expression in mesencephalic dopaminergic neurons of D2 dopamine receptor-deficient mice. *Brain Res Mol Brain Res, 80*(1), 1-6

van Dongen, Y. C., Deniau, J. M., Pennartz, C. M., Galis-de Graaf, Y., Voorn, P., Thierry, A. M., & Groenewegen, H. J. (2005). Anatomical evidence for direct connections between the shell and core subregions of the rat nucleus accumbens. *Neuroscience, 136*(4), 1049-1071. doi: 10.1016/j.neuroscience.2005.08.050

van Rossum, J. M. (1966). The significance of dopamine-receptor blockade for the mechanism of action of neuroleptic drugs. *Arch Int Pharmacodyn Ther, 160*(2), 492-494

Villalba, R. M., Lee, H., & Smith, Y. (2009). Dopaminergic denervation and spine loss in the striatum of MPTP-treated monkeys. *Exp Neurol, 215*(2), 220-227. doi: 10.1016/j.expneurol.2008.09.025

Volkow, N. D., & Baler, R. D. (2014). Addiction science: Uncovering neurobiological complexity. *Neuropharmacology, 76 B*, 235-249. doi: 10.1016/j.neuropharm.2013.05.007

Volkow, N. D., Fowler, J. S., Wang, G. J., Baler, R., & Telang, F. (2009). Imaging dopamine's role in drug abuse and addiction. *Neuropharmacology, 56*, 3-8. doi: 10.1016/j.neuropharm.2008.05.022

Volkow, N. D., Fowler, J. S., Wang, G. J., & Goldstein, R. Z. (2002). Role of dopamine, the frontal cortex and memory circuits in drug addiction: insight from imaging studies. *Neurobiol Learn Mem, 78*(3), 610-624

Volkow, N. D., Fowler, J. S., Wang, G. J., Swanson, J. M., & Telang, F. (2007). Dopamine in drug abuse and addiction: results of imaging studies and treatment implications. *Archives of Neurology, 64*(11), 1575-1579. doi: 10.1001/archneur.64.11.1575

Volkow, N. D., Fowler, J. S., Wang, G. J., Swanson, J. M., & Telang, F. (2007). Dopamine in drug abuse and addiction: results of imaging studies and treatment implications. *Arch Neurol, 64*(11), 1575-1579. doi: 10.1001/archneur.64.11.1575

Volkow, N. D., Wang, G. J., Begleiter, H., Porjesz, B., Fowler, J. S., Telang, F., . . . Thanos, P. K. (2006). High levels of dopamine D2 receptors in unaffected members of alcoholic families: possible protective factors. *Arch Gen Psychiatry, 63*(9), 999-1008. doi: 10.1001/archpsyc.63.9.999

Volpicelli, F., Perrone-Capano, C., Da Pozzo, P., Colucci-D'Amato, L., & di Porzio, U. (2004). Modulation of nurr1 gene expression in mesencephalic dopaminergic neurones. *J Neurochem, 88*(5), 1283-1294

Wedzony, K., Czepiel, K., & Fijal, K. (2001). Immunohistochemical evidence for localization of NMDAR1 receptor subunit on dopaminergic neurons of the rat substantia nigra, pars compacta. *Pol J Pharmacol, 53*(6), 675-679

West, A. E. (2012). Regulated shuttling of the histone deacetylase HDAC5 to the nucleus may put a brake on cocaine addiction. *Neuron, 73*(1), 1-3. doi: 10.1016/j.neuron.2011.12.016

Wichmann, T., & Dostrovsky, J. O. (2011). Pathological basal ganglia activity in movement disorders. *Neuroscience, 198*, 232-244. doi: 10.1016/j.neuroscience.2011.06.048

Wise, R. A. (1987). The role of reward pathways in the development of drug dependence. *Pharmacol Ther, 35*(1-2), 227-263

Wise, R. A. (2009). Roles for nigrostriatal--not just mesocorticolimbic--dopamine in reward and addiction. *Trends in Neurosciences, 32*(10), 517-524. doi: 10.1016/j.tins.2009.06.004

Wolf, M. E., & Roth, R. H. (1990). Autoreceptor regulation of dopamine synthesis. *Ann N Y Acad Sci, 604*, 323-343

Young, K. A., Gobrogge, K. L., & Wang, Z. (2011). The role of mesocorticolimbic dopamine in regulating interactions between drugs of abuse and social behavior. *Neuroscience and Biobehavioral Reviews, 35*(3), 498-515. doi: 10.1016/j.neubiorev.2010.06.004

Zetterstrom, R. H., Solomin, L., Jansson, L., Hoffer, B. J., Olson, L., & Perlmann, T. (1997). Dopamine neuron agenesis in Nurr1-deficient mice. *Science, 276*(5310), 248-250

Vita

Vincent Berry was born in Dearborn, Michigan on September 26, 1988. He attended the University of Michigan-Dearborn from 2007 to 2012 where he earned his Bachelor of Science in Biology and Bachelor of Arts in Philosophy degrees. During his undergraduate career, he volunteered for many clubs and organizations, served as the student body president, and was named as one of the 2012 UM-Dearborn "Difference Makers". Berry went on to complete a Master of Science degree in Medical Sciences from Wayne State University's School of Medicine.

www.ingramcontent.com/pod-product-compliance
Lightning Source LLC
Chambersburg PA
CBHW040252220526
45473CB00001B/451